POCKET GUIDES

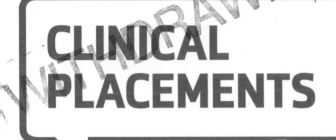

FOR STUDENT NURSES

CLINICAL PLACEMENTS

D0420032

Lantern

ISBN: 9781908625458
First published in 2017 by Lantern Publishing Limited

Lantern Publishing Limited, The Old Hayloft, Vantage Business Park,
Bloxham Road, Banbury OX16 9UX, UK
www.lanternpublishing.com

British Library Cataloguing in Publication Data
A catalogue record for this book is available from the British Library

The authors and publisher have made every attempt to ensure
the content of this book is up to date and accurate. However,
healthcare knowledge and information is changing all the time so
the reader is advised to double-check any information in this text
on drug usage, treatment procedures, the use of equipment, etc.
to confirm that it complies with the latest safety recommendations,
standards of practice and legislation, as well as local Trust policies
and procedures. Students are advised to check with their tutor
and/or mentor before carrying out any of the procedures in this
textbook.

Typeset by Designers Collective Limited
Cover design by Designers Collective Limited
Printed and bound in the UK
Distributed by NBN International, 10 Thornbury Road, Plymouth,
PL6 7PP, UK

Personal information

Name: . . . .

Mobile: . . . .

Address during placement: . . . .

. . . .

. . . .

. . . .

PLACEMENT DETAILS

Hospital: . . . .

Hospital address: . . . .

. . . .

. . . .

. . . .

Link lecturer: . . . .

CONTACT IN CASE OF EMERGENCY

Name: . . . .

Mobile: . . . .

Home/Work number: . . . .

Contents

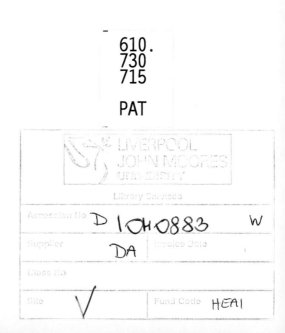

Foreword

Several years ago I was supervising a group of ten second-year nursing students, who were nearing the end of their clinical placement. On our last session I asked them to consider what their top tips would be for those students coming behind them. To my surprise they came up with suggestions which were immensely practical and which I would not have considered: for example, planning bus routes in advance of travelling to placement. Of course they also had tips about clinical issues, such as learning the language of specialist areas: COPD, O_2, IVs, etc., and making friends with Health Care Support Workers (good allies to have on side!). I then asked them as a group to rank their tips on a scale from 1–10. From that exercise we realised that perhaps we were onto something that might benefit students, especially those for whom placement was a new experience. The original "10 top tips" were developed into a conference presentation and subsequently into an article for *Nursing Standard** by myself and two of the ten original students. It was at this point that we were approached to write this book.

*MacDonald, K., Paterson, K. and Wallar, J. (2016) Nursing students' experience of practice placements. Nursing Standard, **31(10)**: 46–51.

Jess and Kirstie have since graduated but have shown great enthusiasm and perseverance in seeing this project through to its completion, especially alongside their postgraduate studies. Both recognise that no matter how experienced you are, starting on a new placement and being a new student again can be a stressful time.

When sharing some of the sections of this book with our current undergraduate students as a means of validating the content, I was reminded once again of how daunting starting a new placement can be. We hope this pocket book will offer some practical advice for students and be a useful reference guide whilst they are in practice.

Kath MacDonald

D.HSSc, MSc, PGCE, Crit. Care Cert.,
Dip. Adv. Nursing, RGN, Nurse Teacher, SFHEA

Senior Lecturer, Division of Nursing, School of Health Sciences
Queen Margaret University, Edinburgh

Acknowledgements

The publishers would like to thank the following students and former students who contributed to the development of this book by reviewing draft outlines and contents. We have listed the universities they were attending during this process, although some of them have graduated and registered as nurses since then, in which case they have survived their placements and congratulations are due!

Suzanne Barke (University of Nottingham)

Harriet Bradfield (University of Cumbria)

Nicole Clinton (Ulster University)

Penny Fawthrop (University of Salford)

Lorna Gallacher (University of Leeds)

Ruth Goddard (Edinburgh Napier University)

Deirdre Mulvenna-Pegrum (University of Surrey)

Abbreviations

A&E	Accident and Emergency	
ABC	airway, breathing, circulation	
ABG	arterial blood gas	
ACE	angiotensin-converting enzyme	
ADLs	activities of daily living	
ALs	activities of living	
ARDS	acute respiratory distress syndrome	
AVPU	alert, verbal, pain, unresponsive	
BLS	basic life support	
BP	blood pressure	
C. diff	*Clostridium difficile*	
CA	cancer	
CD	controlled drug	
CHF	chronic heart failure	
COPD	chronic obstructive pulmonary disease	
CPR	cardiopulmonary resuscitation	
CSU	catheter specimen urine	
CVA	cerebrovascular accident (stroke)	
DNAR	do not attempt resuscitation	
DOB	date of birth	
DVT	deep vein thrombosis	
ECG	electrocardiogram	
ED	emergency department	
ENT	ear, nose, and throat	
ET	endotracheal tube	
GCS	Glasgow Coma Scale	
H_2O	water	
HIV	human immunodeficiency virus	
HR	heart rate	
HTN	hypertension	
I&D	incision and drainage	
I&O	intake and output	
IBS	irritable bowel syndrome	
ICP	intracranial pressure	
ICU/ITU	intensive care unit/intensive treatment unit	
IM	intramuscular	

> Confusion in the use of abbreviations has been cited as the reason for some clinical incidents. Therefore you should use these abbreviations with caution and only in line with local Trusts' Clinical Governance recommendations which vary between departments!

INH	inhaled
IV	intravenous
LOC	level of consciousness
MRSA	methicillin-resistant *Staphylococcus aureus*
MSU	midstream urine specimen
NBM	nil by mouth
NG	nasogastric
NMC	Nursing and Midwifery Council
NSAID	non-steroidal anti-inflammatory drug
O_2	oxygen
O	oral
PE	pulmonary embolism
PPE	personal protective equipment
PR	per rectum
PRN	as needed
PV	per vagina
RBC	red blood cell
SBARD	situation, background, assessment, recommendation, decision
S/C	subcutaneous
S/L	sublingual
SOB	shortness of breath
SPA	suprapubic aspirate
TIA	transient ischaemic attack
TOP	topical
TPN	total parenteral nutrition
TPR	temperature, pulse, respiration
UA	urinalysis
UTI	urinary tract infection
VRE	vancomycin-resistant *Enterococcus*
WBC	white blood cell
WHO	World Health Organization

Getting there

Preparing for placement

ℹ Practical tips

Starting your first placement in the clinical setting will be stressful, but it can also be enjoyable. This pocket guide is intended to take away some of the stress so that you can enjoy your placement and make the most of it.

Your whole routine is about to change and you will be meeting lots of new people. Some tips to think about in advance to help you survive and enjoy placement include:

- Get plenty of rest
- Eat good healthy food
- Keep hydrated throughout the process
- Always remember to ask questions!

✅ Checklist for the week before

☐ Find out the phone number for the ward

☐ Call or visit the clinical area in advance to check

    ☐ what type of unit it is

    ☐ where it is located in the hospital/health centre

    ☐ your shift schedule and the times of your shifts

    ☐ start time on your first day

    ☐ who your mentor is

☐ Arrange travel plans, do a practice run by bus, car or train and remember weekend schedules are different

☐ Find out what the parking costs are if you have a car

☐ Get your uniforms ready and have worn-in comfortable shoes

☐ Ask about changing rooms – they may be located centrally or in the clinical area

☐ Plan what you are going to take for meals and where the staff eat lunch

- [ ] *Find out if you will have access to a microwave and refrigerator*
- [ ] *Buy a water bottle*
- [ ] *Research the clinical speciality of the area you are allocated*
- [ ] *Buy lots of pens and bring this pocketbook with you to write in during your placement*

✓ Checklist of things to bring with you on your first day

- [ ] *Professional practice portfolio (placement documentation from university)*
- [ ] *Your uniform*
- [ ] *Comfortable and appropriate shoes*
- [ ] *Hair ties, if appropriate*
- [ ] *Hand cream and lipbalm*
- [ ] *Water bottle*
- [ ] *This pocket guide*
- [ ] *Enough food for the duration of your shift (more is always better during your first few days to gauge how much is necessary)*
- [ ] *Pens*

 Notes

_____

_____

_____

_____

_____

As a student you will be given the appropriate uniform to wear by your university. Wear your uniform with pride and remember it represents your profession.

Your responsibilities include:

- Hair should be tied back and off the collar (for infection control and to ensure safety, e.g. a confused patient might pull a nurse's hair).
- Nails should be short and clean (no fake, painted or gel nails).
- Always wear your name badge.
- NEVER wear your uniform to and from work. Change in the designated changing rooms at your clinical placement.
- No jewellery or watches should be worn, other than a plain wedding ring or one other plain ring. Jewellery can scratch patients or get caught on something during moving and handling.
- For infection control purposes all undershirts should be above elbow level. If for religious reasons you need to cover your forearms, the clinical area should provide you with disposable sleeve covers.
- Always launder your uniform appropriately and store it correctly.

Remember that these policies are in place to protect our patients and us, as healthcare professionals.

 Your placement may have specific uniform requirements - note them here:

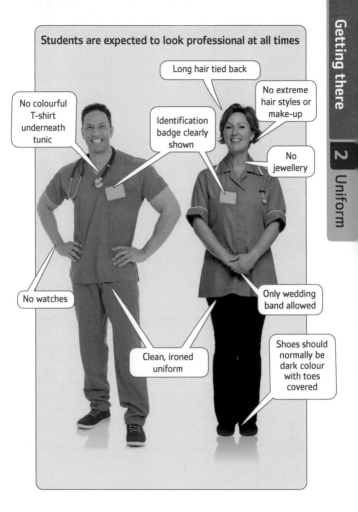

Students are expected to look professional at all times

Long hair tied back

No extreme hair styles or make-up

No colourful T-shirt underneath tunic

Identification badge clearly shown

No jewellery

No watches

Only wedding band allowed

Clean, ironed uniform

Shoes should normally be dark colour with toes covered

Make sure you are aware of the absence policy of both your university and your placement area. Usually this means contacting both areas if for any reason you are unable to attend placement. This is for your own safety – both areas need to know if you have an issue that prevents you attending.

It's also usual to inform both areas when you plan to return. A phone call the day before is enough. If you are absent for more than seven working days you will require a sick note from your GP. You should make a copy of this so that both areas have evidence of your absence.

 Top tip

Check the local absence policy, as policies may vary across placements.

 Notes

4 The NMC Code of Conduct

The Nursing and Midwifery Council (NMC) is the nursing and midwifery regulating body in the UK and provides a Code of Conduct (see our summary below) which contains professional standards that registered nurses and midwives must adhere to. Ensure you are familiar with this before you start your placement. The Code centres around four elements: *prioritising people; practising effectively; preserving safety; and promoting professionalism and trust.*

Prioritise people

- Treat people as individuals
- Help preserve dignity
- Listen to people and respond to their preferences and concerns
- Make sure that people's ever-changing physical and psychosocial needs are being assessed and responded to
- Always act in the best interests of people
- Gain informed consent before carrying out any intervention

  see Section 6: Consent and confidentiality
- Respect people's right to privacy and confidentiality

Practise effectively

- Use evidence-based practice – never do something just because "that's the way we've always done it"
- Communicate effectively with colleagues and patients

  see Sections 11 and 12
- Share your skills and knowledge – let your peers and mentor know if you've read any interesting articles
- Keep clear and accurate records – make sure your mentor or another registered nurse reads and countersigns your notes

Preserve safety

- Recognise and work within the limits of your competence – don't do anything that you're not 100% comfortable doing
- Never give a medicine unless you know what it's for

  see Section 14.2 for tips on safe drug administration

- Be honest if you make a mistake
- Always offer help if an emergency arises in your practice – make sure you know how to call for emergency help in your clinical area
- Make sure you know how to raise concerns if you believe your patient is vulnerable or there is a risk to patient safety

Promote professionalism and trust

- Sometimes patients and their families may not be able to differentiate between a student nurse and a registered nurse. Therefore the way that you conduct yourself is not only important in upholding your own reputation but also the reputation of the nursing profession. Uphold the reputation of your profession at all times – **this applies to when you are studying and in your personal life.**

see *Section 7* for guidance on using social media

Tips for professionalism

- If you're working with a colleague, avoid speaking over or excluding your patient.
- Avoid gossip and topics that demonstrate a lack of professionalism – you are allowed to relax and have a good time off duty, but your patients don't want to hear you saying things like "what a great night last night but did you see the state of that nurse from critical care?"

Make sure that you familiarise yourself with the Code online

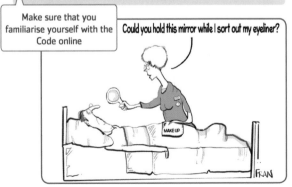

8

Raising concerns

As a student nurse you may witness practice that makes you feel uncomfortable and is not in keeping with the NMC expected professional values of a nurse. Although you may find it difficult to speak out, remember you have a duty of care to your patients. In the first instance discuss this with your mentor or your link lecturer.

> The NMC also has guidance on raising concerns: **bit.do/PG-CP2**

> To make it easy for you to access them, we have shortened web links to this format - simply type these into any web browser and you'll go to the right page!

Notes

_____

_____

_____

_____

_____

_____

_____

Reference: NMC. *The Code: Professional Standards of Practice and Behaviour for Nurses and Midwives.* London, 2015.

Person-centred care (PCC) is a term that will be used throughout your placement. Always ensure your patient is at the centre of their care, include them in decisions and enable them to be a proactive member of the team. As a student nurse you are in a unique position, in that you do not necessarily have the same responsibilities and pressures staff members have. Try to take the time to talk to your patients and learn about the things in their life that matter to them. Treat your patients as you would like your family members or yourself to be treated.

A model that might help you think about PCC is the Person-centred Practice Framework shown opposite. This model has the patient at the centre and is framed by the person-centred processes (the petals on the flower) and surrounded by the organisational systems and prerequisites that are required to be in place to support person-centred processes of care.

 Notes

_____

_____

_____

_____

_____

_____

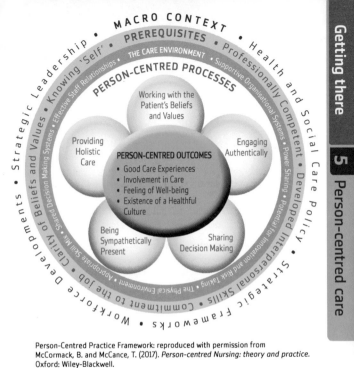

Person-Centred Practice Framework: reproduced with permission from
McCormack, B. and McCance, T. (2017). *Person-centred Nursing: theory and practice.*
Oxford: Wiley-Blackwell.

Notes

The NMC Code reminds us that we must always gain consent before carrying out any intervention. There are three types of consent: written, verbal and implied.

- Written consent is usually required for any invasive procedure, such as a surgical operation, or taking part in a research study.
- Verbal and implied consent are less formal: for example,

> **"Mr Smith, is it OK that I check your blood pressure?"**

Mr Smith may reply "yes", but he may also roll up his sleeve and hold out his arm which illustrates implied consent.

We also need to respect a patient's right to decline treatment – it is important to document if a patient refuses care, for example if they decline a shower or do not consent to have their observations recorded.

We need to treat the information we know about people in our care as confidential – this also means information that they tell you. This is a fundamental element in demonstrating professional conduct, as patients pass on sensitive information to us in confidence.

There are some exceptions to this non-disclosure, such as in the case of vulnerable children or adults, or in relation to communicable diseases. In these cases it's important that you tell the patient that you are not able to keep this a secret.

Ask your mentor or senior nurses on your placement if you have any concerns that you might be breaching confidentiality before engaging in discussion with relatives or unknown health professionals.

Tips on maintaining confidentiality

- Only disclose information to other professionals who are involved in that person's care. Make sure that the information about them is shared appropriately by those who will be providing care. Think – what do they need to know to ensure that care is safe, effective and person-centred?
- Don't speak about patient information in public places – e.g. on the bus home from the hospital! You never know who could be listening.
- Don't take any written information home with you (e.g. patient handover sheets); ensure they are shredded at the end of a shift.
- If for any reason you have to transport records outside the clinical area (e.g. for a home visit), ensure they are in a locked bag and stored in a locked boot if travelling by car.
- When talking to relatives, be careful not to breach confidentiality – it may be helpful to ask them what they have already been told or know about plans for care. Always check with the patient first what information they want shared with friends and relatives.
- A person has a right to confidentiality even after they have died.

 Notes

_____

_____

_____

_____

_____

13

If used appropriately, social networking sites can be beneficial for nurses, midwives and students to build professional relationships and develop support networks – for example through discussion boards – and may provide access to research, clinical experiences and other resources that you didn't know even existed!

It is important that student nurses use personal social media and social networking sites responsibly – you may jeopardise your ability to be registered with the NMC if you act unprofessionally.

Tips on using social media responsibly

- Think before you post – how might this affect your professional registration as a nurse or midwife? Consider the NMC code, even when you are not at work.

- Don't discuss people in your care outside of placement – even if you think that you have anonymised them, other people may still be able to identify them.

- Do not share anything that may be viewed as discriminatory or encourages violence and bullying behaviour – remember to uphold the reputation of the nursing profession at all times.

- Think about your privacy settings – once you've posted something, others may be able to copy and share it further.

- Think about what you "like" or "retweet" and who and what you associate with or which points of view you support. This might imply that you endorse a view that is not in keeping with the values of the NMC code.

- Do not blur professional boundaries with patients by building personal relationships with them – do not "friend" or "follow" patients online – and remember, patients and relatives may still be able to view your profile even if you don't engage with them.
- Think about what you have posted online in the past.
- If you think that another student nurse is using social media in a way that is unprofessional or unlawful then you have a duty of care to report concerns.

Read the NMC document on using social media: Nursing and Midwifery Council (2017). *Guidance on using social media responsibly.* Available at: **bit.do/PG-CP3**

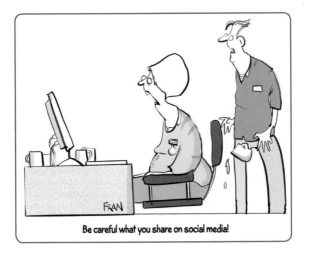

Be careful what you share on social media!

Settling there

Tips for your first day of placement

- Turn up at the agreed time.
- Remember to smile and introduce yourself and ask people for their names and who they are.
- Familiarise yourself with the fire and other emergency protocols (including the numbers to dial, the location of the fire extinguishers and resuscitation trolley).
- Ask for someone to show you around, so you know the layout of the unit and where some key things may be.
- Establish who your mentor(s) will be, and write down their names.
- Verify your allocated shifts on the duty roster to make sure what you have is correct, in addition to the times of the different shifts.
- Be positive and ask questions.
- Leave your mobile phone in your locker and don't use it during shifts except during your break.
- Check how long you have for breaks and don't exceed this.

✎ **Note here the names of as many key colleagues and their roles as you can remember**

_____

_____

_____

_____

_____

_____

_____

_____

_____

_____

Many students are surprised, when starting on placement, that they do not spend all their time "shadowing" their mentor. Remember the NMC standards advise that students should work with their mentor for at least 40% of the time they are in placement.

Supervision can be direct – one-to-one – or at a distance; for example, if your mentor delegates a task to you such as bathing a patient and then "checks in" from time to time.

Your mentor will have other responsibilities during their shift such as co-ordination and bed meetings, so don't expect them to be exclusively yours. Try to sit down with them at the beginning of the placement to discuss both your expectations.

i   Questions to ask your mentor at the start:

- How often will you work with them?
- What do they expect of you?
- How can they help you achieve your objectives?
- What visits would be helpful outside of your area?
- Which other personnel should you work with?
- How will you get your ongoing record of achievement signed off?

During your placement, ask for constructive feedback on your performance – be proactive.

Try to have a discussion with your mentor around the midway mark to discuss what you have achieved and areas for improvement.

If you have concerns about your supervision, talk to your academic link/clinical supervisor. Your university should have a process for raising concerns, and most practice areas have a useful "cause for concern" flowchart, which is a helpful guide to consult in the first instance.

A simple flowchart might look something like this:

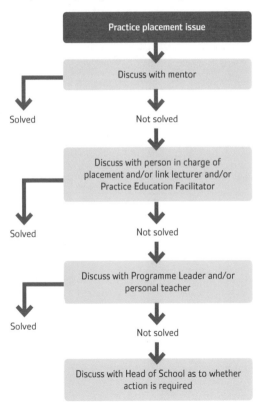

Practice placement issue

Discuss with mentor

Solved ← | → Not solved

Discuss with person in charge of placement and/or link lecturer and/or Practice Education Facilitator

Solved ← | → Not solved

Discuss with Programme Leader and/or personal teacher

Solved ← | → Not solved

Discuss with Head of School as to whether action is required

You should familiarise yourself with the common forms of documentation you will encounter on placement, as shown below. Remember that different locations have different methods of documentation, and many of these may be online. Make sure you are familiar with the documentation used in your placement setting.

Document	Purpose
Drug Kardex	Legal documentation of when the prescribed medications were given to the patient; also provides scheduled times when the medicines must be administered
National Early Warning Scoring System (NEWS) chart; see inside front cover	A standardised approach to the documentation of a patient's vital signs which allocates a score to each of the physiological measurements, e.g. respiratory rate, pulse, oxygen saturation levels, systolic blood pressure and temperature
Datix/critical incident/near miss form	Analyses the error/near miss and the events leading up to it, and how it can be improved in the future
Nursing Kardex (often an electronic patient record, e.g. TRAK in many Scottish Trusts)	Up-to-date nursing documentation of the care that has been delivered

Document	Purpose
Care rounding chart	This documents various interventions and shows the nurse has addressed these. For example, asking the patient if they need the toilet or checking if they have been incontinent or if they need a drink or snack. Frequency varies depending on a patient's needs
Handover sheet	The most up-to-date information on the patients and key information that is necessary for the next shift to have when delivering care
Fluid balance chart (FBC)	A record of fluids in and fluids out; how much was taken by mouth, IV, tube feeding and what was put out, e.g. in urine, faeces, vomit.

 Notes

_____

_____

_____

_____

_____

Communicating with other healthcare professionals can be daunting, especially when you are new in the practice area. Communication breakdown is a leading cause of adverse events in healthcare, so developing your communication skills as a healthcare professional is vital. The SBARD framework shown below is a standardised method of relaying important information effectively and concisely.

Situation	Concise statement of the problem
Background	Pertinent and brief information related to the situation
Assessment	Analysis and considerations of options – what you found/think
Recommendation	Action requested/recommended – what you want
Decision	Action taken

Example of a brief handover scenario from the nurse to a doctor:

S   Ms Brown is a 69-year-old female patient admitted to the hospital for her chronic obstructive pulmonary disease (COPD) exacerbation.

B   Ms Brown uses 2 L of oxygen via nasal cannula at home with regular inhalers. She is an ex-smoker, having quit smoking three months ago. She also has asthma with a history of bronchitis.

A   Her oxygen saturation level is at 85% on 2 L of oxygen via nasal cannula, she is wheezing and very short of breath. She is also anxious.

R   Can her oxygen be increased? What would you like her oxygen saturation levels to be above? Do you think nebuliser treatments could help Ms Brown? Also what about working with physiotherapy for chest physiotherapy? Ms Brown is also asking for something to help with her anxiety.

D   Commence nebulisers, continue 2 L oxygen, start chest physiotherapy.

Tips on answering the phones

Answering the phones in the practice area can be an anxiety-provoking task at first, but the more you do it the more confidence you will have and the more answers you will have to the questions. Here are some tips to help you over the first few calls.

- Pick up, state your name, position, and what unit you are on.
- Simply ask, "What can I help you with?"
- Remember not to disclose any information regarding patients to members of the public, even if they say they are the patient's next of kin.
- Inform the caller that you will get the nurse looking after that patient to speak to them.
- If the caller is another healthcare professional and you feel uncomfortable or don't know the answer to their question, tell them you are a student and will get a member of staff to assist them.

Communication is a skill and it takes time to master. Don't be afraid to ask questions; if you aren't sure of something take the time to stop and ask. You need to feel confident in your learning and practice as a nurse. Your mentor and the nursing team will support you and help you improve your communication skills.

> Make friends with Health Care Support Workers – you can learn a lot from their experiences and knowledge of the clinical environment.

Top tip

Learn any specialist language used in your placement area so you can communicate effectively with colleagues.

Communication is central to everything that nurses do. Poor communication is the commonest reason for complaints in health care. Effective communication can make a positive difference to patients in hospital by ensuring that they feel listened to and supported; and that their concerns are valid, important and acted upon.

Tips for successful communication

- Always introduce yourself by stating your name and role – this identifies you to the patient and their family.
- Ask the patient how they would like to be addressed – Josephine Smith might like being called by her first name (Josephine or Jo), a nickname (such as Sephy or Smithy), or by her title and surname, Mrs Smith.
- Always explain what you are going to do and explain the purpose of the interaction – this may alleviate some anxiety and provides an opportunity to gain informal consent.
- Speak clearly to enhance a patient's understanding – be aware of your tone of voice and the rate at which you speak.
- Choose your words carefully – avoid jargon. Be appropriate for the patient's age and level of understanding. Ask for feedback to ensure that they understand what you want to communicate.
- Consider visual and hearing impairments and language difficulties. For example, a person with a visual impairment may need to be approached from one side only.
- Avoid giving people too much information – this can cause confusion, especially if they have a sensory or cognitive impairment.

- Provide an opportunity to ask questions – this gives the patient a chance to seek clarification and express any concerns.
- Listen **actively** – this is a process whereby we hear what the patient is saying by focusing attention on that patient, through gestures such as head nodding, mirroring what they say and observing their body language.
- Consider the environment in which you are communicating. Factors such as a noisy or busy ward may impede good communication and you may have to find a quiet space to have your conversation, especially if it's confidential.
- Think about your body language and observe the patient's non-verbal communication.
- Good eye contact can help to convey interest. Be mindful of your facial expressions – sometimes there may be smells or sights, or patients might disclose stories to you which might make you feel shocked or disgusted, but it's important that we don't make patients feel uncomfortable.
- Remember: be honest if a patient asks you something and you don't know the answer.

Notes

_____

_____

_____

_____

_____

Being there

13.1 Hand hygiene

i **Top tip**

> Remember that effective hand hygiene is the number one intervention we can make as healthcare professionals to protect our patients from the spread of healthcare-associated infections.

RUB HANDS FOR HAND HYGIENE! WASH HANDS WHEN VISIBLY SOILED

⏱ **Duration of the entire procedure:** 20-30 seconds

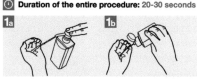

Apply a palmful of the product in a cupped hand, covering all surfaces;

Rub hands palm to palm;

Right palm over left dorsum with interlaced fingers and vice versa;

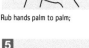

Palm to palm with fingers interlaced;

Backs of fingers to opposing palms with fingers interlocked;

Rotational rubbing of left thumb clasped in right palm and vice versa;

Rotational rubbing, backwards and forwards with clasped fingers of right hand in left palm and vice versa;

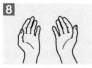

Once dry, your hands are safe.

Proper hand rub technique (World Health Organization, 2009).
Reproduced with permission of the World Health Organization, www.who.int.

Directions for hand washing
(World Health Organization, 2009):

1. Wet hands with water
2. Apply soap
3. Rub hands together (palm to palm)
4. Interlock fingers, alternating hands (palm to palm and top of hand to palm)
5. Back of fingers to opposing palms with fingers interlocked
6. Rub each thumb thoroughly
7. Circular motion of fingertips in opposite palm
8. Rinse hands with water
9. Dry hands thoroughly with a single use paper towel
10. Use towel or elbows to turn off taps

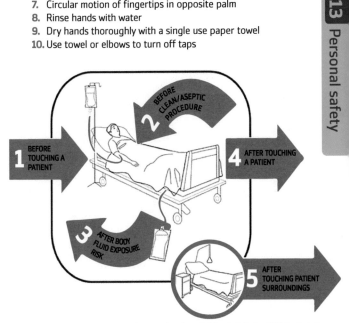

My Five Moments for hand hygiene. Reprinted from *Journal of Hospital Infection*, 67(1), Sax, H. *et al.*, 'My five moments for hand hygiene': a user-centred design approach to understand, train, monitor and report hand hygiene, pp. 9–21 (2007), with permission from Elsevier.

31

If you see someone who does not abide by the proper hand hygiene rules, remember it is our job to advocate for our patients and it is important that we become comfortable asking people to perform hand hygiene. There are different ways to approach this and with more experience you will feel more comfortable confronting colleagues.

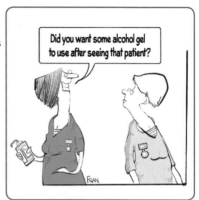

13.2 Infection control and sharps policy

Hospital bins are colour-coded according to the waste that should go in them. It is important to know the colour code and what waste goes in what bin. Here's an example, but check your local policy.

Colour of bin	Use	Example
Black	Domestic waste	Packaging
Yellow	Hazardous and infectious waste	Gloves, aprons, items with blood on
Yellow with black line	Offensive waste	Incontinence pads
Purple	Cytotoxic waste	Chemotherapy drugs
Orange	Infectious waste	Dressings

Confidential information has a specific bin where all the waste will be shredded.

The use of personal protective equipment (PPE) is essential for health and safety (NHS, 2010).

PPE includes: gloves, aprons/gowns, face protection, mouth/eye protection.

Often there are colour-coded aprons/gowns for various activities; see below. For example, a certain colour is used for serving food and another is used for patient care activities. Ensure that the gowns are changed at the necessary times, i.e. between tasks or patients.

Activity	Apron or gown	Gloves	Face, eye/mouth protection
Contact with intact skin	N/A	N/A	N/A
Sterile procedures	Yes	Yes	Risk assessment
Contact with wounds, skin lesions	Yes	Yes	Risk assessment
Potential exposure to blood/other body fluids	Yes	Yes	Risk assessment
Handling specimens	Yes	Yes	N/A
Using disinfectants, cleaning agents	Yes	Yes	Risk assessment
Bed making, dressing patients	Yes	Risk assessment	N/A
Oral care	Risk assessment	Yes	Risk assessment
Feeding a patient	Yes	Risk assessment	N/A
Handling waste	Risk assessment	Yes	Risk assessment

Sharps bins

- Any sharp instruments must be placed in a yellow/orange 'sharps bin' after use, for incineration (a purple sharps bin is for cytotoxic waste and there are designated bins for disposing of glass).
- Remember to always have a sharps bin within reach when handling sharp materials such as a needle, in order to dispose of the instrument immediately.
- Always clean up your own sharps, and never someone else's sharps.
- Never re-sheath a needle.

Tips for if you get a needle-stick injury

- Tell your mentor or someone you are working with.
- Wash the cut immediately with running water while milking the wound to make it bleed.
- Cover as applicable.
- Contact Occupational Health for follow-up. They will be able to instruct you on the necessary steps and whether you need blood tests/vaccinations, based upon the type of exposure.
- Never be afraid of telling someone you made a mistake and need help. Your safety should be your priority.
- File an incident report depending on policy in your placement area (remember policies may vary between areas).

 Notes

_____

_____

_____

13.3 Moving and handling

Musculoskeletal injuries such as back pain are a serious problem within the nursing profession so it is essential that we use approved techniques when we are moving and handling patients. This helps to protect both patients and ourselves from injury.

Assessing risk with TILE

Before carrying out any moving and handling task, whether you are helping a patient get out of bed or need to carry a box, you must always assess risk.

Task	What do you want to do/achieve? e.g. assist the patient out of bed.
Individual	What are your individual capabilities? Consider your own health – for example, do you have any existing health conditions or injuries, are you pregnant? Consider the abilities of your colleagues who may also be involved.
Load	This refers to the patient or object. Additional equipment may be required, e.g. manual handling aids, additional pillows, sliding sheets, hoists.
Environment	Consider the space/environment that you are working in – you may have to remove any potential hazards.

 Notes

_____

_____

_____

Factors to consider before you begin moving a patient:

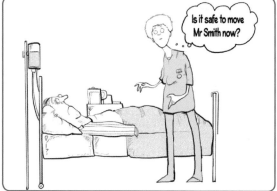

- Is this the right time to move this patient? For example, do they need pain relief before moving and has enough time passed for the analgesia to take effect?
- Am I carrying out this task/movement in the correct way?
- Is the patient fully weight-bearing?
- Does the patient have any weakness? Will they need additional support, e.g. pillows to maintain their position?
- Is the patient wearing appropriate footwear to move?
- Does the patient have a walking aid that should be used?
- Do I need another person to help me assist the patient to move?
- Is the environment safe? Do I need to declutter the immediate area to make the environment safe?
- Does the patient have any devices in place such as a catheter, drain or IV fluids? Have I made sure that they are safely positioned before movement?
- How can I ensure dignity is maintained?
- Have I communicated with the patient and explained what is about to happen?

Tips on moving a patient

- Think about your own body position when moving and handling patients, objects and equipment.
- Continuously assess personal and patient risks.
- If a patient looks like they are about to fall – don't catch them or try to keep them up. Assist them to the floor if it is safe to do so and seek help.
- If a patient falls, do not attempt to lift them off the floor manually. Either the patient will get up independently with some guidance, or a hoist (or other appropriate equipment) should be used to raise the patient.
- If you're unsure about how to move any patient, seek advice from your mentor or colleagues – including your placement area's physiotherapist.
- Always remember to communicate with the patient and explain what you are doing.

If you witness or are made to perform incorrect moving and handling procedures, depending on your level of confidence you could either:

- address the situation as it occurs by suggesting alternative methods and using the necessary equipment; or if you feel uncomfortable
- discuss the situation with your mentor, charge nurse, and/or your clinical supervisor after the event occurs.

Remember the principles behind correct moving and handling procedures and never do anything that could cause harm to a patient or to yourself.

WHO (2009) *SAVE LIVES: Clean Your Hands*. Available at: bit.do/PG-CP4

NHS Professionals (2010). *Standard Infection Control Precautions*. Available at: bit.do/PG-CP5

14.1 Assessment using activities of living

Nurses can use, for example, the twelve activities of living of the Roper–Logan–Tierney model of nursing to assist in the initial assessment of a new patient and to identify any specific needs the patient may have from the activities engaged in, regardless of age and health status.

Activities of living, or ALs, are also referred to as "activities of daily living", or ADLs.

1. Maintaining a safe environment
Nurses must minimise risk to patient safety wherever possible. Examples of actions taken to help maintain a safe environment include: effective hand hygiene to prevent the spread of infection, ensuring that any spills are wiped up and that fire exits are always clear and faulty equipment is reported to the appropriate person.

2. Communication
Consider the patient's cognitive and perceptual abilities and whether they require additional support to aid communication. For example, do they wear glasses or hearing aids or use a speech aid, and are there any potential language or cultural barriers?

see *Section 12* for more tips on communicating with patients.

3. Breathing
Assess respiratory pattern, rate, depth and effort as discussed in *Section 14.4*. Consider if the patient has an underlying respiratory condition such as chronic lung disease (COPD) or asthma. Establish if the patient smokes – if appropriate, this may be a good health-promoting opportunity to discuss smoking cessation.

4. Eating and drinking

Consider the patient's daily food intake. Do they have a good appetite? Do they have any strong likes or dislikes? Do they have a special diet, any food allergies or take additional nutritional supplements? Establish whether the patient can eat independently or requires any assistance with eating and drinking, or if they use adapted cutlery.

5. Elimination

Consider what the patient's normal bowel and urinary habits are. For example, do they experience constipation or do they wake up in the night to urinate (nocturia)? Do they ever experience incontinence? Some patients may require assistance when going to the toilet – it's important to establish what is normal for them so that we can help them to maintain and promote their independence as much as possible in hospital.

6. Washing and dressing

Establish the level of assistance, if any, required for the patient to meet their hygiene needs. Some people may only require additional assistance to carry out fine motor movements such as shaving or doing up buttons.

7. Controlling temperature

Is the patient's temperature within normal range? Are they feeling hot or cold or shivering or sweating? Consider any factors which may influence temperature; for example, in the presence of infection, the administration of antipyretic medications may help reduce a high temperature.

8. Mobilisation

Establish if your patient requires any assistance or mobility equipment to walk or mobilise. Consider if they are at risk of falling or if they have a history of falling.

9. Working and playing

Work provides a sense of purpose and, for many, pride. Find out about current or previous roles and responsibilities. The patient may be worried about the financial implications of being in hospital or whether they will be able to return to work without any problems. Find out about any hobbies or interests the patient may have, as this can provide stimuli for meaningful conversation and help to reduce stress and anxiety whilst they are in hospital.

10. Expressing sexuality

In addition to sexual function, this encompasses the patient's own perceptions of their body image, roles with their family and relationships.

11. Sleeping

Consider sleeping and rest patterns. Note any reasons for variation or disruptions (e.g. emotional or physical problems) and whether the patient requires additional aids to help them sleep, for example medication or a milky drink.

12. Death and dying

This element of the activities of living is not always obvious in nursing assessment or care planning. However, death is inevitable. Although the patient in your care may not be dying, thoughts of death and dying can naturally occur during an admission to hospital, or memories of the death of a family member or friend may be evoked.

Establish what the patient knows about their health condition and what the plan of care is. Does the patient have an advance directive (sometimes called a living will)? If the patient has multiple morbidities and poor quality of life, check their Do Not Actively Resuscitate (DNAR) order. The patient should be fully aware of this (unless they have no intellectual capacity) and this should be recorded in the medical and nursing notes.

14.2 Drug administration

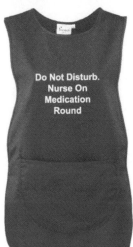

Do Not Disturb.
Nurse On
Medication
Round

"Do not disturb" tabards are often worn by nurses during drug rounds to minimise interruptions and avoid drug errors.
Image supplied courtesy of Kova Manufacturing Ltd, Birmingham.

Administering medication is an important role of the nurse (see the *Five "Rights" of drug administration*, over the page). The skill and professional judgement involved in drug administration is essential in improving patient safety and reducing drug and prescription errors.

The "Right"	Action
Right patient	Check the identity of the patient on the prescription and the patient – ask them to identify themselves by stating full name and date of birth or check identity of patient against their wristband including their unique hospital number. Confirm patient's allergy status.
Right medicine	Check the prescription and that it matches the medication label. Check that the medicine is within expiry date.
Right dose	Check the prescription that the correct dose has been prescribed – you may need to check by calculating the dose.
Right route	Check that the prescribed route is appropriate and that the patient can take/receive the medication by this route.
Right time	Check the frequency of medicine administration and that it is prescribed for the correct time; confirm when the last dose was given (including any once-only doses administered earlier).

Routes of administration

Enteral: this route uses the gastrointestinal (GI) tract for absorption of medicines – examples include oral administration (tablets, liquids) which is swallowed or via a feeding tube such as a nasogastric tube.

Inhaled: e.g. nasal sprays and inhalers.

Parenteral: this route bypasses the GI tract e.g. injections.

Injection: types of injections are:

- subcutaneous (medicine goes into the fatty tissue beneath the skin)
- intramuscular (medicine goes into muscle)
- intravenous injection/infusion (into vein)
- intravesical (directly into the bladder)
- intrathecal (directly into the central nervous system).

Mucous membrane routes: medicines which are not absorbed by the GI tract and are instead applied to the mucous membranes, e.g. vaginal, rectal, buccal (medicine is held against the inside of the cheek); sublingual (dissolves under the tongue).

Topical: medicines which are not absorbed by the GI tract and are instead applied to the skin, e.g. creams, ointments, transdermal patches.

Less common routes: intra-arterial (into artery supplying the organ); intra-articular (into the joint).

Abbreviation	Meaning
IV	Intravenous
IM	Intramuscular
S/C	Subcutaneous
O	Oral
S/L	Sublingual
TOP	Topical
INH	Inhaled
PR	Per rectum
PV	Per vagina

Controlled drugs

- Controlled drugs (CDs) are drugs which are classified under the Misuse of Drugs Act (1971), e.g. morphine.
- They must be stored in a locked cupboard.
- The nurse in charge is responsible for the controlled drug key – this can be delegated to another registered nurse.
- Each clinical area has a controlled drug book which keeps a record of controlled drugs received from pharmacy and the administered controlled drug.
- Regular stock checks are carried out by two registered nurses to ensure that the stated balance of the book reflects the contents of the stock cupboard.
- Two registered nurses are involved in the administration of a controlled drug. First the stock needs to be compared against the balance of the book. Then one person takes the drug out of the cupboard, prepares the prescribed dose and administers the drug. The second person is the checker. These roles should not be interchangeable during this process.
- All entries in the controlled drug book must be signed by a registered nurse and witnessed by a second registered nurse.
- **Student nurses can also be one of the two people required in the administration of a controlled drug – check your university's policy and hospital Trust policy regarding this, as institutions vary with regard to which year you can start participating in this.**
- Entries into the controlled drug book include: name of patient; date and time of administration, dose and quantity administered (and quantity discarded if applicable e.g. if only 5 ml of a 10 ml vial is required); name and signature of person administering the drug; name and signature of person witnessing process; the balance of stock remaining.
- As with any skill, make sure that you are comfortable with the process of administering a controlled drug before you participate.

Tips for administering drugs

- Be certain of the patient's identity and check whether the patient has any allergies before you administer medication.
- Patients with an allergy should wear a red identity band marked with any drug allergens.
- Never give a medicine unless you know what it's for – some medicines are used for more than one condition so check the *British National Formulary* (BNF) to make sure it's the right dose.
- Sometimes prescribers' handwriting can be hard to read, making it difficult to tell exactly what medicine has been prescribed – get the prescriber to rewrite the prescription and confirm this before administering the medication.
- Sign for any medicine you have administered immediately to reduce risk of a drug error – but ensure that the patient has taken the medicine before you sign for it.
- Don't leave medicines by the bed if the patient isn't there.
- Document reasons why medications were not administered – for example, if a patient refuses – according to local policy.

> Student nurses must never administer medication without direct supervision – both the student and registered nurse must sign the medication chart.

 Notes

_____

_____

_____

14.3 Drug calculations

Administering medication is a task nurses perform many times every day so it is essential that you can calculate medicine dosages accurately and confidently.

Like all skills, this is a skill that takes a lot of time and practice to develop so take every opportunity to practise! There are lots of sample questions in *Numeracy and Clinical Calculations for Nurses*; see *Section 23*.

Tablets and capsules

$$\text{No. of tablets} = \frac{\text{What you want (dose prescribed)}}{\text{What you've got (dose per tablet/capsule)}}$$

Example

400 mg of ibuprofen is prescribed. The stock dosage is 200 mg. How many tablets should be given?

400 mg/200 mg = 2 tablets

Liquids and syrups

$$\text{Volume to be given} = \frac{\begin{array}{c}\text{What you want}\\ \text{(dose prescribed) x volume of liquid}\end{array}}{\begin{array}{c}\text{What you've got}\\ \text{(dose of drug in stated volume)}\end{array}}$$

Example

250 mg of paracetamol is prescribed. The stock dosage is in liquid form of 500 mg/10 ml. How many millilitres should be given?

250 mg/500 ml x 10 = ½ x 10 = 5 ml

Unit	Abbreviation	Equivalent	Abbreviation
1 kilogram	kg	1000 grams	g
1 gram	g	1000 milligrams	mg
1 milligram	mg	1000 micrograms	mcg*
1 microgram	mcg	1000 nanograms	ng*
1 litre	L or l	1000 millilitres	ml
1 mole	mol	1000 millimoles	mmol
1 millimole	mmol	1000 micromoles	mcmol

*It is recommended that micrograms and nanograms should never be abbreviated

Conversions

Sometimes the prescribed dose and the stock dose are different. The dosage calculation should be worked out in the same unit so that they are still the same strength.

Example

Convert 0.5 milligrams into micrograms

- Micrograms are smaller than milligrams so multiply by 1000
- Therefore, 0.5 milligrams x 1000 = 500 micrograms

Convert 500 micrograms into milligrams

- Milligrams are bigger than micrograms so divide by 1000
- Therefore, 500 micrograms/1000 = 0.5 milligrams

> Do the calculation in your head first, or written down on paper – then check with a calculator.

 Top tip

If the answer looks wrong – e.g. if the number looks very large – double-check it; do the calculation again! Remember, student nurses only administer medication under the direct supervision of a registered nurse so ask your mentor for help!

14.4 Observations – National Early Warning Score (NEWS)

As a student nurse you will often be asked to take a set of vital signs on patients. It is important to spend time with your mentor and ask any questions if you are unsure of how to do something. It sounds obvious, but do not make up numbers! If you aren't sure how to take a measurement, always ask. Most of the components can be measured using an appropriate machine. However, if possible, check a manual reading if it doesn't feel right to you and if the results are not within the normal range for that patient.

This is the order of the main vital signs as laid out by the NEWS chart (see inside front cover).

Respiration rate:
* Count for a minute how many breaths your patient takes. Remember that if you tell them what you are doing, they may subconsciously change their breathing frequency or pattern.
* A normal respiration rate is between 12 and 20 respirations per minute.

Oxygen saturation level:
* When assessing this component it is also important to record if the patient is on any oxygen or if they have any past medical history that may pertain to their results (i.e. COPD, etc.).
* Peripheral oxygen saturation (SpO_2) is an estimation of the oxygen saturation level, usually measured with a pulse oximeter. A normal SpO_2 is in the range 94–99% (on air).
* Colour – is the patient's skin pink, or is there a blue tinge to the lips, tongue or nails? (implies lack of oxygen).

Blood pressure:
- Always check that you are using the correct blood pressure cuff on a person before taking the measurement, either manually or by a machine.
- Large or very small arms may need a non-standard cuff.
- If you are unhappy with a reading check the other arm for comparison.

Heart rate:
- This is often checked with the vital signs machine.
- It is also a good idea to check the pulse manually in order to feel for the strength, regularity and rate.

ACVPU (alert, confusion, verbal, pain, unresponsive):
- Check the patient's neurological status.
  Are they responding properly to you?
- Has the patient's mental state changed? Do they show new signs of confusion, disorientation or delirium?
- Are they responsive to verbal stimulation, pain stimulation or simply unresponsive?

Temperature:
- Double-check a temperature reading if the patient's temperature is outside the normal range or if the thermometer appears faulty.
- If a patient is recording a very low temperature (e.g. hypothermia), a core (rectal) temperature may be required after checking another thermometer.

Familiarise yourself with the NEWS chart on the inside front cover of this guide, and always ask your mentor or a registered nurse questions if you are not sure how to complete it properly.

Remember: if vital signs are not within normal range it is important that you inform your nurse or the responsible registered nurse, as you are working under their delegation.

Reference: Royal College of Physicians. *National Early Warning Score (NEWS) 2: Standardising the assessment of acute-illness severity in the NHS.* Updated report of a working party. London: RCP, 2017. Available at: bit.do/PG-CP19

14.5 Skin assessment

Pressure sores/ulcers are an area of localised tissue damage caused by excess pressure applied directly to the skin, shearing and/or friction.

They can be painful, prolong hospital stay, become infected and (in extreme cases) be a contributing factor in a patient's death.

What are the risk factors for developing pressure sores?
- Age (older people)
- Immobility or reduced mobility
- Malnutrition
- Loss of sensation – patients with reduced sensation might not be able to alter their position themselves, so it's important to check skin for any redness or signs of skin breakage
- Vascular disease
- Existing restrictions, injuries or recent surgery
- Moisture on skin, e.g. incontinence and excessive perspiration
- Ill-fitting equipment aids which do not provide appropriate pressure relief.

Signs of pressure ulcer/sore development – look out for:
- Persistent erythema (redness)
- Non-blanching erythema – this means that when pressed, the area does not turn white
- Blisters
- Skin may appear shiny or discoloured
- Localised heat
- Localised oedema (swelling)
- Vulnerable areas: heels, sacrum, elbows, back of skull, shoulders, toes.

Top tip

> In patients with darker skin, the affected area of skin may appear purplish/bluish.

Waterlow

The Waterlow scale is an example of a structured scoring tool used to identify people at risk of developing pressure sores whilst in hospital (see inside back cover). It involves assessing the patient's skin and identifying additional factors which may increase a patient's overall risk of developing a pressure ulcer. Other tools are available, e.g. Braden risk assessment tool.

Patients who are identified as being more vulnerable to skin breakdown will be encouraged or assisted to change their position regularly. Manual handling aids such as specialist mattresses and cushions can be used to relieve pressure by evenly redistributing the weight of a patient.

14.6 Urinalysis

The analysis of urine can provide us with important information about a patient's health which can assist in the diagnosis of medical conditions. It can also help us monitor the progression of disease and effects of treatment.

Methods of collecting urine
- Natural voiding into a specimen pot.
- Transfer of urine from bedpan/urinal into a specimen pot.
- Midstream urinalysis (MSU) – genitals must be cleaned to reduce presence of contaminants such as bacteria. Ask the patient to pass urine into the toilet and then catch the middle part of the flow of urine into a sterile container and then pass the remaining urine into the toilet.
- A pad – some clinical areas have kits to enable a urine sample to be collected from an incontinence pad when a patient is unable to follow the above collection methods. The process involves placing a small sterile pad into a clean continence pad. Once the patient has urinated, the pad can be squeezed and a syringe can assist in aspirating the sample. The kit has detailed instructions for use, including the maximum duration that the testing pad can be left in place.

- Catheter specimen of urine (CSU) – clean sampling port of catheter with alcohol-based swab and allow it to dry for 30 seconds. If using a needle-less system, insert syringe into port and aspirate urine (approximately 10 ml). Some ports may require a needle and syringe. Insert needle into port at 45° angle, aspirate and remove needle. Sometimes there isn't enough urine in the catheter tubing to extract, so you may have to clamp the tubing to allow enough urine to accumulate for collection. Remember to unclamp the tubing afterwards to allow drainage to continue.
- Suprapubic aspirate (SPA) – a doctor or advanced nurse practitioner will collect a sterile sample of urine by inserting a needle into the patient's bladder just above the pubic bone.
- 24-hour urine collection – used to assess kidney function by collecting and assessing urine collected over a 24-hour period.

Physical appearance

Before using a dipstick (reagent) test to analyse urine, consider the colour, clarity and smell of the sample.

 Notes

_____

_____

_____

_____

_____

_____

Colour	
Light yellow or straw colour	Normal
Dark yellow	May indicate patient is dehydrated
Bright red or reddish-brown	May suggest blood in the urine (haematuria)
Brown–green or strong yellow	May suggest bilirubin is present, which can be indicative of liver or gall bladder problems
Clarity	
Clear	Normal
Cloudy or containing small particles of debris	May be due to presence of pus, protein or white blood cells, which can be indicative of infection, kidney stones or urinary stasis
Smell	
Very little smell	Normal
'Fishy' smell	May indicate presence of infection, or that a sample has been waiting too long to be tested – a sample should be tested within 2 hours of collection
Sweet or fruity smell	May suggest presence of ketone bodies which are by-products of fat metabolism and may indicate patients who have been fasting or have diabetic hyperglycaemia (see table overleaf)

 Top tip

Some foods and medications can produce certain smells (e.g. asparagus) or can alter the colour of urine (e.g. beetroot).

Urine analysis

Reagent strips are a quick, easy and non-invasive way of testing urine. It is important that you understand what the findings mean so that you can report any abnormalities to your mentor – see below.

Test	Normal value	Common cause of change
Leucocytes	Not usually found in urine	The presence of leucocytes is an indication of a renal/bladder urinary tract infection (UTI)
Nitrates	Not usually found in urine	Presence suggests a UTI
Protein	Normal urine has low levels of the proteins albumin and globulin which are not enough to give a positive reagent strip reaction	High levels may suggest UTI, renal conditions, heart failure, pre-eclampsia
pH	4.5–8.0	Low pH (strongly acidic, pH <4) may be caused by diabetes, starvation and dehydration High pH (alkaline, pH >8) may indicate stale urine which is unsuitable for further testing
Blood (haematuria)	Not usually found in urine	Haematuria may suggest renal or urinary tract conditions

Look out for a false positive if a female is menstruating

Test	Normal value	Common cause of change
Specific gravity Tests the concentration and diluting abilities of the kidneys	1.005–1.030	High concentration may indicate dehydration Low concentration indicates very dilute urine which may be because of a high fluid intake or may be caused by renal abnormalities
Ketones Ketones are produced by the breakdown of fatty acid	Not usually found in urine	These may be present because of fasting (e.g. vomiting) or uncontrolled diabetes
Glucose	Not usually found in urine	Presence may be associated with raised blood glucose (diabetes), pregnancy and renal abnormalities

Tips for urinalysis

- Before you begin urinalysis, check the expiry date of the reagent strips and make sure that the container hasn't been left open.
- Wash your hands before and after – always wear gloves.
- Use a fresh urine sample to ensure the best results.
- When removing the strip from the urine sample, run the edges of the strip against the container or a paper towel to remove excess urine.
- Hold reagent strip close to the colour blocks on the bottle of the reagent strips to match carefully.
- Wait for the time recommended by the urinalysis reagent strips, to ensure accurate results.
- Record the results and report any abnormalities to your mentor or a staff nurse.

Roper N., Logan W.W. & Tierney A.J. (2000). *The Roper–Logan–Tierney Model of Nursing: Based on Activities of Living*. Edinburgh: Elsevier Health Sciences

Waterlow (2007) The Waterlow Assessment Tool. Available at: bit.do/PG-CP17

If you come across an unresponsive or choking patient in your clinical placement remember to shout for help and that you are never alone. Assess the situation for your own safety first and then intervene. Never do anything that you are not confident of or that puts your own safety at risk.

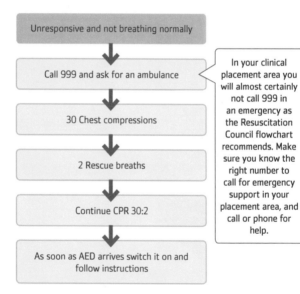

Adult Basic Life Support (Resuscitation Council, 2015).
CPR 30:2 – an emergency cardiopulmonary resuscitation procedure that alternates 30 chest compressions with two rescue breaths; AED – automated external defibrillator (a portable device that checks the heart rhythm and can send an electric shock to the heart to try to restore a normal rhythm). Reproduced with the kind permission of the Resuscitation Council (UK).

```
                    ┌──────────┐
                    │  Assess  │
                    │ severity │
                    └──────────┘
            ┌──────────┴──────────┐
            ▼                     ▼
    ┌───────────────┐     ┌───────────────┐
    │    Severe     │     │     Mild      │
    │Airway obstruction│  │Airway obstruction│
    │(ineffective cough)│ │(effective cough)│
    └───────────────┘     └───────────────┘
     ┌─────┴─────┐               ▼
     ▼           ▼       ┌───────────────────┐
```

Unconscious	Conscious	Encourage cough
Start CPR	5 back blows 5 abdominal thrusts	Continue to check for deterioration to ineffective cough or until obstruction relieved

Adult choking guidelines (Resuscitation Council, 2015). Reproduced with the kind permission of the Resuscitation Council (UK).

If you need to start CPR see the Adult Basic Life Support algorithm, opposite.

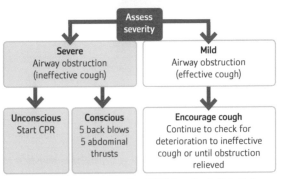

- Always keep the airway opened by tilting the head back (head tilt, chin lift).
- Do not put anything in the patient's mouth.
- Wait for help before moving the patient.
- If it is safe to do so, or no neck injury is apparent, place in the recovery position.
- Time and record events as they happen.

The recovery position. Reproduced from *Clinical Skills for OSCEs*, 5th ed. © Neel Burton, 2015.

Resuscitation Council (2015) Resuscitation guidelines. Available at: bit.do/PG-CP18

16.1 Anaphylactic reaction

Anaphylaxis is a severe, potentially life-threatening allergic reaction.

- Patients having a reaction should be assessed and treated using the Airway, Breathing, Circulation, Disability, Exposure (ABCDE) approach.
- Most reactions occur quite quickly after exposure to an allergen. Signs of an anaphylactic reaction are:
  - patient is very anxious
  - airway swelling (tongue swelling, difficulty breathing and swallowing, feeling like their throat is closing)
  - shortness of breath
  - wheezing
  - patient is pale and/or clammy
  - tachycardia
  - hypotension
  - decrease/loss of consciousness
  - cardiac arrest.
- If necessary, depending on the patient's condition, carry out basic life support (see *Section 15*).
- The patient's treatment plan will vary according to their location and the cause of the allergy.
- If an anaphylactic reaction occurred during medication administration/blood transfusion, make sure the IV is switched off.
- After an anaphylactic reaction patients should be referred to an allergy specialist.
- Intramuscular adrenaline is regarded as the treatment of choice (if a patient has a known allergy, to peanuts for example, they should carry their EpiPen at all times).
- Document in the notes what happened, the time and what action was taken.

16.2 Falls

Falls are the second most common cause of accidental or unintentional injury and death worldwide, after road traffic injuries (WHO, 2016).

- Fall prevention is a priority in nursing to provide a safe environment. Preventative measures include:
  - screening
  - identifying predisposing risk factors (e.g. low blood pressure, medications)
  - home assessments
  - use of assistive devices (e.g, walking sticks, frames)
  - muscle strengthening, balance exercises, etc.
- Care rounding involves environmental checks for the patient to ensure all preventative measures against falls are taken. For example:
  - check the patient has the necessary footwear
  - ensure good organisation of IV lines
  - declutter the patient's bed space
  - ensure the patient has everything they need within reach, including their call bell
  - if the patient is confused or impulsive consider a chair/bed alarm.
- Before you move a patient always check with the nurse or physiotherapist on what equipment is required and how the patient mobilises. If you are ever in doubt have another person with you. If you are walking/transferring a patient and they begin to fall do not try to catch them but if safe to do so try to cushion their fall to the ground without hurting yourself (see *Section 13.3* for information on moving and handling patients).

If a patient has fallen:

- Make sure the patient is safe and call for help.
- Check their vital signs and assess any injuries (e.g. if they hit their head or have any other obvious signs of injury).
- Depending on the patient's level of ability, use moving and handling equipment to slowly help the patient up. The patient should first get on their knees and then stand up if they are able to.
- Inform the doctor of the patient's fall and ask what else they would like you to do.

In the event of a fall, write an incident report explaining what happened, as per the local policy in the clinical area. Also document the event in the nursing progress notes, stating the time of the fall, the vital signs after the fall, the orders from the doctors and other information pertinent to the specific situation.

 Top tip

> Learning how to document incident reports as a student nurse is important, so ask to work with your mentor to complete this task.

✐ **Notes**

16.3 Sepsis

Sepsis	Severe sepsis	Septic shock
• body temperature >38°C or <36°C • heart rate >90 beats/minute • respiratory rate >20 breaths a minute or $PaCO_2$ <32 mmHg • white blood cell count >12 000 or <4000 mm^3 or >10% band forms	• decreased urine output • change in mental status • decrease in platelet count • difficulty breathing • abdominal pain • abnormal heart beating	• signs and symptoms of severe sepsis and hypotension despite adequate fluid replacement

- To be diagnosed as having sepsis a patient must present with at least two of the symptoms of sepsis listed in the table above.
- Early identification is key in reducing mortality.
- Different types of infection can cause sepsis; however, the most common causes are:
  - pneumonia
  - abdominal infection
  - kidney infection
  - blood stream infection.
- This may all seem overwhelming to you as a student nurse and you may not know what it all means but you **must** remember to inform your mentor of abnormal vital signs as it could be an indication that the patient may have sepsis.
- The NEWS assessment tool helps healthcare professionals identify the possibility that a patient may have sepsis (see *Section 14.4* and inside front cover).

16.4 Stroke

Does something seem not right with your patient? Are you concerned? Complete this quick assessment for stroke using FAST:

Face	Does their face droop to one side? Can they smile?
Arms	Can they raise both arms and keep them there?
Speech	Is their speech slurred?
Time	Quickly alert the doctor if any of these signs of stroke are present. Note the time.

Time is critical, so alert the nurse you are working with immediately if you are concerned or have noticed any symptoms that could indicate a stroke. Once the doctors are aware they will order more tests/scans to assess the patient and determine the treatment plan.

Transient ischaemic attack

A TIA or transient ischaemic attack (also known as a mini-stroke) is the same as a stroke, except that the symptoms last for a short amount of time and no longer than 24 hours. The FAST test can be used to recognise the signs of TIA as well. Don't wait to see if the symptoms pass or get better.

Although the symptoms may not last long, a TIA is still very serious. It's a warning sign that a person is at risk of going on to have a stroke.

WHO (2016). Falls. Available at: bit.do/PG-CP11

17

Common groups of medications

Medication should not be prescribed by trade name; rather it should always be in the generic form.

Reason for medication (commonly referred to as)	Medication group	Medication name (not an exhaustive list)
Pain relief	Analgesics	Paracetamol, ibuprofen, co-codamol, codeine, tramadol and morphine sulphate
Nausea	Anti-emetic	Metoclopramide, ondansetron, promethazine hydrochloride, cyclizine
Cholesterol-reducing	Statins	Atorvastatin, simvastatin, lovastatin
Blood thinner	Antiplatelet drugs, anticoagulants	Rivaroxaban, aspirin, heparin, warfarin
Water pill	Diuretic	Furosemide, bendroflumethiazide
Itch/allergy	Antipruritic	Antihistamines (diphenhydramine), corticosteroids (topical (e.g. betamethasone) and oral (e.g. prednisone))
Lowers blood pressure	Antihypertensive	Calcium channel blockers (amlodipine), ACE inhibitors (lisinopril, ramipril), beta-blockers (atenolol, metoprolol)
Bacterial infection	Antibiotics	Penicillins (amoxicillin), erythromycin, clarithromycin, azithromycin, ciprofloxacin, levofloxacin, vancomycin, metronidazole

Constipation	Laxatives	Docusate, senna, suppositories, polyethylene glycol, milk of magnesia
Irregular heartbeat	Anti-arrhythmics	Digoxin

 Notes

_____

_____

_____

_____

_____

_____

_____

_____

_____

_____

18

Pain assessment – pain tools

Pain is subjective and experienced differently by everyone. It can be physical and emotional.

Type of pain	Duration	Examples
Acute	<12 weeks	Surgery, trauma, acute disease or illness Brief duration
Chronic	>12 weeks	Neuropathic pain e.g. back pain
Malignant	Pain associated in patients with advanced cancer/metastatic cancer	
Referred	Pain is experienced away from the affected area; e.g. pain may originate from the heart but is experienced in the back, neck and jaw	

Tips for assessing pain

Talk to the person – listen to the words they use to describe their pain

Words often used to describe pain include:

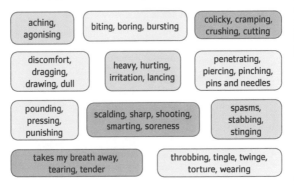

aching, agonising

biting, boring, bursting

colicky, cramping, crushing, cutting

discomfort, dragging, drawing, dull

heavy, hurting, irritation, lancing

penetrating, piercing, pinching, pins and needles

pounding, pressing, punishing

scalding, sharp, shooting, smarting, soreness

spasms, stabbing, stinging

takes my breath away, tearing, tender

throbbing, tingle, twinge, torture, wearing

> Effective communication skills are fundamental for effectively assessing and managing pain. Think about your patient's age, culture, cognitive abilities and any communication difficulties that they might have.

Some questions that may help you to understand the person's pain:

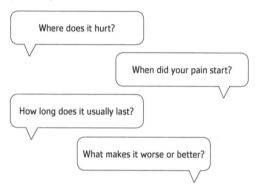

Where does it hurt?

When did your pain start?

How long does it usually last?

What makes it worse or better?

Pain assessment tools

Numerical rating scale (NRS) – the patient chooses a number on the scale which best describes their pain. Zero represents no pain at all, whereas a score of 10 represents the worst pain imaginable.

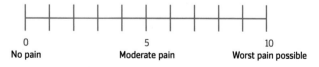

0	5	10
No pain	Moderate pain	Worst pain possible

Verbal rating scale (VRS) provides graded categories: "no pain", "slight pain", "moderate pain", "very bad pain" and "agonising pain".

Make sure the tool you use is appropriate for the individual and their age, cognitive/developmental ability and level of understanding. It may be better to use a visual tool, as shown below.

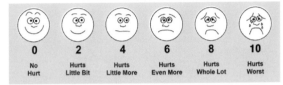

0	2	4	6	8	10
No Hurt	Hurts Little Bit	Hurts Little More	Hurts Even More	Hurts Whole Lot	Hurts Worst

Wong–Baker FACES® Pain Rating Scale. Reproduced with permission from the Wong–Baker FACES Foundation.

 Notes

Pain management

If a patient's pain is not managed effectively, this can slow down their recovery. There are two approaches to managing pain – pharmacological and non-pharmacological.

Pharmacological means using drugs e.g. paracetamol, ibuprofen, codeine, morphine (see *Section 17*).

Non-pharmacological approaches include complementary and alternative therapies, such as acupuncture, aromatherapy and reflexology, and transcutaneous electrical nerve stimulation (TENS), where low voltage electricity is applied to the body via electrodes.

Art and music therapy, hypnosis, use of imagery, distraction including conversation, watching TV or reading a book are other non-pharmacological approaches to pain management.

 Top tip

> Try to arrange some time with your placement area's pain team and find out more!

Moving on from there

Nurses who reflect have a better understanding of their experiences and this can help them to continue to develop their skills and enhance their nursing knowledge. Therefore it is essential that nursing students learn to reflect during their programme.

Reflection is something that we do naturally without even thinking about – it's a way of considering and reviewing our experiences and feelings, evaluating what went well or what didn't go so well and considering what could be done differently next time.

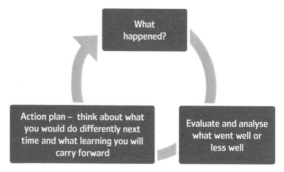

What happened?

Action plan – think about what you would do differently next time and what learning you will carry forward

Evaluate and analyse what went well or less well

Trigger questions for reflection.

Reflection can be structured or unstructured and can be an individual or group activity. Examples of structured reflection include:

- reflective essay writing
- group reflective sessions led by a facilitator during clinical practice.

Gibbs' Reflective Cycle and Oelofsen's three-stage CLT model (curiosity, looking deeper, transformation) are examples of useful frameworks that can help structure reflection.

> That session with Mrs Macdonald went really well today. I wonder why that was?

> What did I do that contributed? What alternatives might I have considered? What else do I need to know to support my development in this area?

> What would I do differently next time to make it even better?

Unstructured reflection can happen naturally through conversation with your mentor or discussion with friends. Some students may also like to explore their experiences through other creative outlets such as poetry (e.g. haikus), story-telling or writing in personal journals.

> **A haiku:**
> Learnt new skills today
> Vital signs, medications
> Time to reflect now

Top tip

Remember to respect patients' right to confidentiality and to anonymise them if you are talking to friends or if you are writing down your experiences.

Gibbs, G. (1988) *Learning by Doing: a guide to teaching and learning methods*. Oxford: Oxford Polytechnic Further Education Unit.

Oelofsen, N. (2012) *Developing Reflective Practice: a guide for health and social care students and practitioners*. Banbury: Lantern Publishing Ltd.

What should I do if I witness substandard care of a patient?

It depends on the severity of the situation; however, there are different ways that you could handle such a case. If you feel comfortable you could talk to the charge nurse in the clinical setting and/or discuss the situation with your clinical supervisor (point of contact with your university). Also, you can discuss the scenario with your fellow classmates (ensuring confidentiality is upheld). You have a duty of care to share this information with someone more senior.

What happens if I make a mistake in practice?

It is important that you tell someone in practice as soon as possible that you have made the mistake. It may be something minor; however, if it is more serious an incident form may have to be filed. It is important that you discuss this in clinical supervision and a meeting may be arranged with your clinical supervisor and mentor/charge nurse from clinical practice.

What should I do if I don't feel comfortable doing something?

Always speak your mind and let the people you are working with know that you aren't comfortable. Don't be afraid to ask questions. Remember that you are supernumerary and should not feel that you are obliged to perform a task, especially if you did not receive the necessary directions/information and feel uncomfortable.

What should I do if my feet keep hurting and I generally feel run down?

It is really important that you buy comfortable and supportive shoes. Get enough sleep, eat well-balanced meals, stay hydrated and ask for support/advice from your colleagues. Try to maintain a good work/life balance and try not to think about your placement when you are off duty; keep up with friends/family and hobbies.

How can I look after myself following an emergency situation?

Normally there will be a debrief after a stressful event in practice. Ask any questions that you feel are pertinent to the situation. It may be useful to keep a journal and write down some of the feelings you have after your first emergency situation. Perhaps it could be used for a reflective account for university. Read up on the patient and research any information that is unfamiliar to you, so that if this situation were to arise again in the future you would have the necessary skills and experience to feel more prepared.

What happens if I am not enjoying my placement? Or I don't like my mentor?

Try to make the most of each placement. Even if you feel you are not learning as much as you could be, organise different experiences to enhance your placement and get the most out of it. Never be afraid of asking to see different aspects of the patient's care; for example, going to the operating theatre, spending time with specialist nurses, attending multidisciplinary team meetings and working with other members of the team.

5Rs	right patient; right medicine; right dose; right route; right time
ADLs	activities of daily living e.g. walking, personal hygiene, nutrition and hydration, sleeping patterns, skin assessment, perception of self, sexuality (including body image and family roles); also known as activities of living
Afebrile or apyrexial	absence of fever
Anuria	absence of urine production
Atrophy	wasting
Bradycardia	low heart rate (<60 beats per minute)
Diuresis	voiding large amounts of urine
Dysphagia	difficulty swallowing
Dysphasia	difficulty speaking
Dyspnoea	difficulty breathing
Dysrhythmia, arrhythmia	abnormal heartbeat

Dysuria	painful urination
Erythema	redness
Excoriation	raw surface
Haematemesis	blood in vomit
Haematuria	blood in urine
Haemoptysis	blood in sputum
Hyperglycaemia	high blood sugar (>11 mmol/L)
Hypoglycaemia	low blood sugar (<4 mmol/L)
Necrosis	death of tissue
Nocturia	frequent urination overnight
Oliguria	decreased urine output
Orthopnoea	difficulty/inability to breathe while lying down
Palliative	to alleviate symptoms
Polyuria	excessive urine
Prophylactic	preventative
Pruritus	itching
Tachycardia	fast heart rate (>100 beats per minute)

The table below shows normal vital sign ranges and blood glucose parameters (adults).

Respiratory rate	12–20 breaths per minute
Pulse rate	60–100 beats per minute
Blood pressure range	100/60 – 140/80 mmHg
Blood glucose	4–7 mmol/L

The following table gives metric units and their equivalents.

Unit	Abbreviation	Equivalent	Abbreviation
1 kilogram	kg	1000 grams	g
1 gram	g	1000 milligrams	mg
1 milligram	mg	1000 micrograms	mcg*
1 microgram	mcg	1000 nanograms	ng*
1 litre	L or l	1000 millilitres	ml
1 mole	mol	1000 millimoles	mmol
1 millimole	mmol	1000 micromoles	mcmol

*It is recommended that micrograms and nanograms should never be abbreviated

Common medical emergencies

Macintosh, M. and Moore, T. (2011) *Caring for the Seriously Ill Patient,* 2nd ed. London: Hodder Arnold, pp. 128–9.

Mayo Clinic (2017) *Sepsis.* Available at: bit.do/PG-CP6

NICE (2013) *Falls: assessment and prevention of falls in older people* (CG161). Available at: bit.do/PG-CP7

NICE (2016) *Anaphylaxis.* Available at: bit.do/PG-CP8

Resuscitation Council (2008). Emergency treatment of anaphylactic reactions. Available at: bit.do/PG-CP9

Society of Critical Care Medicine (2016) *Surviving Sepsis Campaign: Guidelines.* Available at: bit.do/PG-CP10

WHO (2016) *Falls.* Available at: bit.do/PG-CP11

Communication

Blom, L., Petersson, P., Hagell, P. and Westergreen, A. (2015) The Situation, Background, Assessment and Recommendation (SBAR) model for communication between health care professionals: a clinical intervention pilot study. *International Journal of Caring Sciences,* 8(3): 530–5.

hello my name is... campaign: http://hellomynameis.org.uk/

Institute for Healthcare Improvement (2017) *SBAR.* Available at: bit.do/PG-CP12

Pavord, E. and Donnelly, E. (2015) *Communication and Interpersonal Skills.* Banbury: Lantern Publishing Limited.

Vlitos, K. and Kamara, S. (2016) Improving communication of important information using the SBARD tool. *Mental Health Practice,* 20(2): 34–8.

Fundamental skills

CSP (2014) *Guidance in Manual Handling for Chartered Physiotherapists,* 4th ed. London: Charted Society of Physiotherapy.

Davison, N. (2015) *Numeracy and Clinical Calculations for Nurses.* Banbury: Lantern Publishing Limited.

Dougherty, L., Lister, S. and West-Oram, A. (2015). *The Royal Marsden Manual of Clinical Nursing Procedures: student edition,* 9th ed. Chichester: Wiley-Blackwell.

Federico, F. (2011) *The 5 Rights of Medication Administration.* Available at: bit.do/PG-CP13

Health Improvement Scotland (2009) Braden Risk Assessment Tool. Available at: bit.do/PG-CP14

McDonald, W., Ness, V., Taylor, K., McGuinness, C. and Simpson, E. (2009) Chapter 2: Mandatory skills. In *Foundation Clinical Nursing Skills,* ed. C. Docherty and J. McCallum, pp. 5–112. Oxford: Oxford University Press.

NMC (2010) *Standards for Medicines Management.* Available at: bit.do/PG-CP15

Spires, A. and O'Brien, M. (2011) *Introduction to Medicines Management in Nursing.* Exeter: Learning Matters.

Medications

BNF Publications (2017) *British National Formulary.* Available online via MedicinesComplete at: www.bnf.org/

Pain

British Pain Society www.britishpainsociety.org.uk

Chamley, C. (2011) Chapter 19: Pain management. In *Alexander's Nursing Practice,* 4th ed., ed. C. Brooker and M. Nicol, pp. 551–73. Edinburgh: Churchill Livingstone.

Department of Health (2010) *Essence of Care: benchmarks for the prevention and management of pain.* Available at: bit.do/PG-CP16

All websites accessed 1 August 2017

Notes

Notes

Notes

Notes